THE WEIGHT LOSS REVOLUTION

Breakthrough Treatments and Lifestyle Strategies for Rapid Weight Loss

BY

DR. MICHAEL GAMBACORTA

THE MEDICAL WEIGHT LOSS REVOLUTION

Breakthrough Treatments and Lifestyle Strategies for Rapid Weight Loss

To my wife,

You are the heart behind every success we've achieved together.

Without your unwavering strength, dedication, and partnership, our shared vision would have never become a reality.

Your brilliance, compassion, and endless support have been the cornerstone of everything we've created.

To our incredible family—Cole and Lex—you are the reason for everything we do.

Your love, resilience, and spirit inspire me daily.

With all my love and gratitude,

Michael

ABOUT THE AUTHOR

Dr. Michael Gambacorta is a healthcare innovator blending traditional and alternative medicine to provide comprehensive care. As the owner and lead physician at Myrtle Beach Spine Center, he focuses on Physical Medicine and Rehabilitation, specializing in the treatment of spinal conditions and musculoskeletal health. His unique approach is shaped 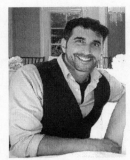 by dual expertise—being both a Family Nurse Practitioner (board-certified in family medicine) and a Chiropractic Physician. This combination allows him to offer a holistic treatment model that addresses both the symptoms and root causes of his patients' health issues.

Dr. Gambacorta's academic career is as extensive as his professional one. He earned his Doctor of Chiropractic degree from Logan University and graduated Summa Cum Laude from Herzing University, where he became a Family Nurse Practitioner. Additionally, his nursing education from the International College of Health Science saw him recognized as a member of the prestigious Sigma Theta Tau National Honors Society. His journey in healthcare started with a Bachelor's degree in Biology from Canisius College, where he was also a Division-1 collegiate soccer player.

Throughout his career, Dr. Gambacorta has founded and led several successful ventures. He is the owner of Myrtle Beach Regenerative Medicine, offering cutting-edge treatments for chronic pain and injury recovery, and the newly established Medical Weight Loss 4-You, focusing on sustainable and medically supervised weight loss solutions. His entrepreneurial spirit first shone through as the founder of the Goldsboro Spine Center (2004-2018) and Capri Day Spa (2012-2021).

In addition to his clinical work, Dr. Gambacorta is an accomplished author with two books to his name: "Longevity: The Future of Healthcare" (2021) and "The Healthy Alternative" (2011). These publications reflect his dedication to educating the public about proactive and integrative approaches to health.

His passion for leadership is evident through his Executive Certification in Leadership, Management, and Negotiation from Notre Dame University. His athletic and academic achievements earned him a place in the Lewiston-Porter High School Hall of Fame in 2020.

Dr. Gambacorta holds numerous professional certifications, including EMG/NCV from Tufts University School of Medicine, Diagnostic Ultrasound guided injections, and Radiology, further enhancing his ability to diagnose and treat complex medical conditions. He is also First Responder Certified and CPR Certified by the American Heart Association. With a deep commitment to patient care, Dr. Gambacorta continues to push the boundaries of medical innovation, offering solutions that improve the quality of life for his patients. His clinical expertise, entrepreneurial success, and dedication to integrative healthcare make him a respected leader in the field.

CONTENTS

CHAPTER 1: Prescription Medications for Medical Weight Loss and Beyond   1

CHAPTER 2: Bariatric Surgery - Understanding the Options and Implications   3

CHAPTER 3: Metabolic Rate and Hormonal Balance - The Drivers of Fat Storage and Weight Loss   11

CHAPTER 4: Nutritional Counseling - Creating Tailored Diets for Lasting Weight Loss and Health   19

CHAPTER 5: Behavioral Therapy - Cognitive-Behavioral Approaches for Changing Eating Habits and Emotional Eating   29

CHAPTER 6: Exercise Prescription - Structured Programs for Fat Loss, Muscle Preservation, and Metabolic Health   37

CHAPTER 7: Gut Health & Microbiome - The Influence of Gut Bacteria on Weight Management   47

CHAPTER 8: Medical Conditions & Weight - Addressing Challenges in Weight Loss with Hypothyroidism, PCOS, and Diabetes   55

CHAPTER 9: Long-Term Weight Management - Sustaining Weight Loss and Promoting Longevity   63

CHAPTER 10: Insurance Coverage for Weight Loss Treatments - Navigating Health Insurance for Medications, Surgeries, and Counseling for Obesity   71

"The greatest wealth is health."

– VIRGIL

CHAPTER 1

Prescription Medications for Medical Weight Loss and Beyond

Introduction

In recent years, prescription medications like semaglutide, tirzepatide, liraglutide, and phentermine have transformed the landscape of medical weight loss. Initially developed for conditions like diabetes, these medications have found broader use in combating obesity and related health issues. This chapter will explore these medications, how they work, their benefits, side effects, and other off-label uses. We will also dive into the latest trends and research supporting their efficacy.

Semaglutide (Ozempic/Wegovy)

Semaglutide is a glucagon-like peptide-1 (GLP-1) receptor agonist, primarily used to manage type 2 diabetes. Marketed under the names Ozempic (for diabetes) and Wegovy (for weight loss), it has garnered attention for its potent effects on weight management.

Mechanism of Action

Semaglutide mimics the action of the GLP-1 hormone, which is naturally secreted in response to food intake. GLP-1 slows gastric emptying, stimulates insulin secretion, and decreases glucagon levels, leading to better blood sugar control. By making people feel fuller longer, it naturally reduces calorie intake, which helps with weight loss.

Efficacy and Research

In clinical trials, semaglutide has shown remarkable results. A study published in the *New England Journal of Medicine* (Wilding, et al., 2021) demonstrated that participants using Wegovy lost an average of 15-20% of their body weight over 68 weeks compared to placebo groups. This level of weight loss is unprecedented for a drug treatment, rivaling bariatric surgery outcomes.

Benefits

- **Substantial weight loss:** Wegovy has been proven to induce significant, sustained weight loss in obese patients.
- **Blood sugar control:** Ozempic is highly effective for diabetes management, lowering HbA1c levels in type 2 diabetes patients.
- **Cardiovascular benefits:** Studies suggest GLP-1 receptor agonists like semaglutide reduce cardiovascular risks, including stroke and heart attack, in high-risk individuals.

Side Effects

Common side effects include nausea, vomiting, diarrhea, and constipation, usually as the body adjusts to the drug. Some patients report severe gastro-intestinal distress, particularly at higher doses. There is also a concern over an increased risk of thyroid tumors, which was observed in animal studies, though this has not been definitively shown in humans.

Tirzepatide (Zepbound)

Tirzepatide (marketed as Zepbound for weight loss and Mounjaro for diabetes) is a dual glucose-dependent insulinotropic polypeptide (GIP) and GLP-1 receptor agonist. By targeting both GIP and GLP-1 receptors, tirzepatide offers a unique mechanism for both glycemic control and weight reduction.

Mechanism of Action

Tirzepatide not only mimics GLP-1 but also GIP, another hormone involved in glucose regulation and fat metabolism. This dual action leads to more efficient insulin secretion, enhanced satiety, and improved fat metabolism.

Efficacy and Research

Tirzepatide has shown to be even more effective than semaglutide. In the *SURMOUNT-1* trial, patients using Zepbound lost an average of 20.9% of their body weight, with some achieving reductions over 25%. This positions tirzepatide as one of the most powerful pharmaceutical tools for obesity management.

Benefits

- **Enhanced weight loss:** Tirzepatide appears to outperform other GLP-1 medications in promoting significant fat loss.
- **Dual action:** The combination of GIP and GLP-1 pathways enhances its overall effectiveness in both diabetes and obesity treatment.
- **Insulin sensitivity:** The drug improves insulin sensitivity, reducing insulin resistance in patients with type 2 diabetes.

Side Effects

As with other GLP-1 agonists, common side effects include nausea, diarrhea, and vomiting. Some patients may experience fatigue and low blood sugar, especially when used alongside insulin or sulfonylureas. Gastrointestinal side effects tend to diminish over time.

Liraglutide (Saxenda)

Liraglutide is another GLP-1 receptor agonist, available under the brand names Saxenda (for weight loss) and Victoza (for diabetes). Liraglutide has a shorter half-life than semaglutide, requiring daily injections rather than weekly.

Mechanism of Action

Like semaglutide, liraglutide slows gastric emptying, reduces appetite, and increases insulin secretion. While effective, its impact on weight loss is somewhat less dramatic than semaglutide or tirzepatide.

Efficacy and Research

Clinical trials have shown that Saxenda leads to an average weight loss of around 8-10% over 56 weeks, a significant improvement compared to diet and exercise alone. A study published in *The Lancet* (Pi-Sunyer et al., 2015) found that liraglutide reduced body weight by 8.4% on average in obese patients without diabetes.

Benefits

- **Moderate weight loss:** Liraglutide provides consistent, though somewhat less dramatic, weight loss compared to newer agents.
- **Diabetes management:** Victoza effectively lowers blood sugar and reduces the risk of cardiovascular events in patients with diabetes.
- **Daily dosing:** While some may see this as a drawback, daily injections allow for better control over side effects and dose adjustments.

Side Effects

Side effects are similar to other GLP-1 agonists, including nausea, vomiting, and gastrointestinal discomfort. Some patients report more frequent headaches and dizziness compared to semaglutide or tirzepatide.

Phentermine

Phentermine is one of the oldest and most well-known medications for short-term weight loss. It is a sympathomimetic amine that stimulates the central nervous system, reducing appetite and increasing energy expenditure.

Mechanism of Action

Phentermine acts as an appetite suppressant by increasing the release of norepinephrine in the brain, leading to reduced hunger and increased energy. It is typically prescribed for short-term use (12 weeks or less) due to its potential for dependency and cardiovascular side effects.

Efficacy and Research

Phentermine, while effective, does not offer the same level of weight loss as GLP-1 or GIP/GLP-1 receptor agonists. A study in *Obesity Reviews* (Yanovski & Yanovski, 2014) found that patients lost around 5% of their body weight with phentermine over 12 weeks. While effective for short-term weight loss, the results are less sustainable without lifestyle changes.

Benefits

- **Rapid weight loss:** Phentermine can kickstart weight loss in patients struggling to lose weight through diet and exercise alone.
- **Increased energy:** Many users report higher energy levels and motivation to engage in physical activity.
- **Low cost:** Phentermine is often much cheaper than newer weight loss drugs, making it more accessible for those without insurance coverage.

Side Effects

Common side effects include dry mouth, insomnia, dizziness, and increased heart rate. Due to its stimulant effects, phentermine can cause dependency, and long-term use is generally discouraged.

Off-Label Uses and Emerging Trends

Beyond weight loss and diabetes, GLP-1 agonists and tirzepatide are being studied for a variety of off-label uses. These include:

▸ **Polycystic Ovary Syndrome (PCOS):** GLP-1 agonists have shown promise in improving insulin sensitivity and reducing weight in women with PCOS.

▸ **Non-alcoholic fatty liver disease (NAFLD):** Emerging research suggests GLP-1 medications may help reduce liver fat and inflammation.

▸ **Addiction treatment:** GLP-1 agonists are being investigated for their potential role in reducing cravings for alcohol and nicotine.

Conclusion

The use of medications like semaglutide, tirzepatide, liraglutide, and phentermine has revolutionized the field of medical weight loss. With ongoing research and a growing understanding of their benefits and risks, these drugs offer new hope for those struggling with obesity, diabetes, and other related conditions. However, patients must weigh the potential side effects and long-term sustainability of these treatments alongside their benefits. As these drugs continue to evolve, they may find even broader uses in managing a wide range of health conditions.

"Take care of your body.
It's the only place you
have to live."

– JIM ROHN

CHAPTER 2

Bariatric Surgery
Understanding the Options and Implications

Introduction

Bariatric surgery, or weight-loss surgery, has become one of the most effective treatments for severe obesity when lifestyle interventions such as diet, exercise, and medication have failed. Procedures like gastric bypass, sleeve gastrectomy, and lap band surgery are designed to reduce stomach size, limit food intake, and, in some cases, alter digestion. While bariatric surgery can lead to substantial weight loss and health improvements, it is a major life change that comes with significant risks, side effects, and long-term considerations. In this chapter, we will explore the different types of bariatric surgery, the people who can benefit, the risks involved, and how life is impacted after surgery.

Prevalence and Candidates for Bariatric Surgery

Obesity continues to be a major public health crisis, affecting over 42% of adults in the United States according to data from the Centers for Disease Control and Prevention (CDC). For those with severe obesity (BMI ≥ 40) or individuals with a BMI ≥ 35 and obesity-related conditions like type 2 diabetes or hypertension, bariatric surgery has become an increasingly common treatment option. According to the American Society for Metabolic and Bariatric Surgery (ASMBS), approximately 250,000 bariatric surgeries were performed in the U.S. in 2021 alone. Globally, over 600,000 bariatric surgeries are performed each year, with the number steadily rising as obesity rates increase.

Candidates for bariatric surgery are typically individuals who:

- Have a BMI ≥ 40, or a BMI ≥ 35 with serious health conditions such as type 2 diabetes, sleep apnea, or heart disease.
- Have failed to achieve lasting weight loss through diet, exercise, and medical treatments.
- Are willing to commit to long-term lifestyle changes, including dietary adjustments, exercise, and regular medical follow-ups.

Types of Bariatric Surgery

There are several types of bariatric surgery, each with its own mechanism and risk profile. The most common procedures include:

- Roux-en-Y Gastric Bypass (RYGB)
- Sleeve Gastrectomy
- Adjustable Gastric Banding (Lap Band)

Roux-en-Y Gastric Bypass (RYGB)

Gastric bypass surgery is one of the most widely performed and effective bariatric surgeries. In this procedure, a small stomach pouch is created by dividing the upper stomach, which is then connected directly to the small intestine, bypassing a large portion of the stomach and part of the intestines. This significantly reduces the amount of food the stomach can hold and alters the digestive process.

Benefits

- **Significant and rapid weight loss:** Patients can lose 60-80% of their excess body weight within 18-24 months.

- **Improvement of comorbidities:** Conditions such as type 2 diabetes, high blood pressure, and sleep apnea often improve or resolve after surgery.
- **Long-term success:** Gastric bypass tends to offer durable, long-term weight loss with many patients maintaining a reduced body weight for over a decade.

Risks and Complications

- **Dumping syndrome:** This occurs when food moves too quickly from the stomach to the small intestine, leading to symptoms such as nausea, vomiting, diarrhea, and dizziness.
- **Nutritional deficiencies:** Since part of the intestine is bypassed, patients can experience malabsorption of essential nutrients like iron, calcium, vitamin B12, and folate. Lifelong vitamin and mineral supplementation is often necessary.
- **Surgical risks:** As with any major surgery, there is a risk of infection, blood clots, and complications related to anesthesia.

Sleeve Gastrectomy

Sleeve gastrectomy is currently the most popular bariatric procedure in the U.S. and involves removing about 75-80% of the stomach, leaving behind a tube-like "sleeve." This reduces the stomach's capacity and lowers levels of the hunger hormone ghrelin, resulting in reduced appetite.

Benefits

- **Significant weight loss:** Patients typically lose 50-70% of their excess body weight within 18 months.
- **Simpler procedure:** Unlike gastric bypass, sleeve gastrectomy does not involve rerouting the intestines, which reduces the risk of complications like dumping syndrome and malabsorption.

> ▸ **Improved metabolic health:** Many patients see rapid improvements in conditions like type 2 diabetes and hypertension.

Risks and Complications

> ▸ **Nutritional deficiencies:** While less severe than gastric bypass, patients may still require lifelong supplementation for vitamins and minerals, particularly iron, calcium, and vitamin D.
> ▸ **Gastroesophageal reflux disease (GERD):** Some patients experience worsened acid reflux or develop GERD after surgery.
> ▸ **Leakage:** There is a small risk of leakage along the stapled portion of the stomach, which can lead to serious infections.

Adjustable Gastric Banding (Lap Band)

Lap band surgery involves placing an adjustable silicone band around the upper part of the stomach to create a small pouch. The size of the band can be adjusted by inflating or deflating a saline-filled balloon inside the band, which can be done through a port placed under the skin.

Benefits

> ▸ **Less invasive:** Unlike sleeve gastrectomy or gastric bypass, no part of the stomach or intestines is removed or rerouted, and the procedure is reversible.
> ▸ **Gradual weight loss:** Patients generally lose 40-50% of their excess weight over two to five years.
> ▸ **Lower surgical risk:** Because the procedure is less invasive, there are fewer risks related to surgery itself, such as infections or internal bleeding.

Risks and Complications

▸ **Slower weight loss:** Weight loss with the lap band is generally slower and less significant than other types of bariatric surgery.

▸ **Band slippage or erosion:** The band can slip or erode into the stomach over time, requiring additional surgeries.

▸ **Frequent adjustments:** Patients must visit their doctor regularly for band adjustments, which can be time-consuming and costly.

Who Can Benefit from Bariatric Surgery?

Bariatric surgery is not a one-size-fits-all solution. It is most beneficial for individuals who have struggled with obesity for years and have been unable to lose weight through conventional methods. The following groups may see the most benefit from surgery:

▸ **Individuals with severe obesity (BMI ≥ 40):** These individuals are at high risk for obesity-related conditions like type 2 diabetes, heart disease, and sleep apnea, and bariatric surgery can reduce these risks by promoting significant weight loss.

▸ **Individuals with obesity-related health conditions (BMI ≥ 35):** For those with a BMI of 35-39.9, bariatric surgery is often recommended if they have serious conditions like type 2 diabetes, high blood pressure, or severe arthritis.

▸ **Patients with a strong support system:** Successful outcomes are often dependent on a patient's ability to adhere to the necessary lifestyle changes post-surgery. A strong support network of family, friends, and healthcare providers can increase the likelihood of long-term success.

Life After Surgery: What to Expect

The decision to undergo bariatric surgery is life-changing, not just in terms of weight loss but in how one lives day to day.

Immediate Post-Operative Recovery

▶ **Dietary changes:** In the weeks following surgery, patients must follow a strict diet, starting with liquids and gradually progressing to pureed foods, soft foods, and eventually small, solid meals.

▶ **Pain and discomfort:** Some degree of pain, swelling, and discomfort is expected after surgery, though this is usually manageable with prescribed medications.

▶ **Activity:** Patients are encouraged to begin light physical activity as soon as possible to prevent blood clots and promote healing, though heavy lifting and strenuous exercise are off-limits for several weeks.

Long-Term Lifestyle Changes

▶ **Dietary restrictions:** Patients must permanently adopt new eating habits, including eating smaller, more frequent meals, chewing food thoroughly, and avoiding high-fat, high-sugar foods that can trigger dumping syndrome (in gastric bypass patients).

▶ **Vitamin supplementation:** Since bariatric surgery alters the digestive system, many patients require lifelong vitamin and mineral supplementation to avoid deficiencies.

▶ **Regular follow-ups:** Patients will need to schedule regular follow-up appointments with their healthcare provider to monitor progress, adjust medications, and address any nutritional deficiencies or complications.

Long-Term Complications

While bariatric surgery can result in significant health benefits, there are potential long-term complications that patients need to be aware of:

- ▶ **Nutritional deficiencies:** As mentioned earlier, patients are at risk for deficiencies in vitamins and minerals such as iron, calcium, vitamin D, and vitamin B12, which can lead to conditions like anemia, osteoporosis, and neuropathy.
- ▶ **Weight regain:** Although bariatric surgery promotes rapid weight loss, some patients may regain weight over time due to factors such as stretching of the stomach pouch, poor dietary habits, or lack of physical activity.
- ▶ **Surgical revisions:** Some patients may require additional surgeries to correct issues such as stomach pouch stretching, hernias, or band slippage (in lap band patients).
- ▶ **Psychological effects:** Significant weight loss can lead to body image issues, excess skin, and emotional stress. Some patients may experience depression, anxiety, or difficulties adjusting to their new body.

Conclusion

Bariatric surgery is a powerful tool in the fight against severe obesity, offering substantial weight loss and improvement in health conditions like diabetes and heart disease. However, it is not without risks, and it requires a lifelong commitment to dietary changes, exercise, and medical monitoring. For those who are unable to lose weight through traditional methods, bariatric surgery can be life altering, it is often advised to try all available methods of weight loss first before undergoing bariatric surgery.

"Those who think they have no time for healthy eating will sooner or later have to find time for illness."

– EDWARD STANLEY

CHAPTER 3

Metabolic Rate and Hormonal Balance

The Drivers of Fat Storage and Weight Loss

Introduction

The body's metabolic rate and hormonal balance are essential components in weight regulation, fat storage, and overall health. Metabolism refers to the process by which the body converts food into energy, and it can vary significantly between individuals due to genetics, age, and activity levels. Hormones, on the other hand, act as messengers that regulate a variety of bodily functions, including hunger, energy use, and fat storage.

Key hormones like insulin, leptin, cortisol, and thyroid hormones play pivotal roles in determining how the body processes and stores fat. This chapter will explore the connections between metabolism and these hormones, how imbalances can contribute to weight gain, and natural methods to improve thyroid and cortisol function to promote fat loss and better health.

Understanding Metabolism and Basal Metabolic Rate (BMR)

Basal Metabolic Rate (BMR) refers to the number of calories your body needs to maintain basic physiological functions while at rest, such as breathing, digestion, and regulating body temperature. BMR is influenced by several factors, including age, gender, muscle mass, and hormone levels. The higher the BMR, the more calories the body burns at rest, making it easier to lose or maintain weight.

Metabolic rate, in general, is affected by:

- ▶ **Muscle mass:** Muscle burns more calories than fat tissue, even at rest.
- ▶ **Age:** As we age, BMR tends to slow down due to loss of muscle mass and hormonal changes.
- ▶ **Hormonal balance:** Hormones like thyroid hormone, insulin, and cortisol directly influence how efficiently your body burns calories and stores fat.

When metabolism is functioning efficiently, the body uses energy from food effectively and maintains a healthy weight. However, metabolic dysfunction often results in weight gain or difficulty losing weight.

The Role of Thyroid Hormones in Metabolism

The thyroid gland, located in the neck, produces hormones that regulate metabolism. The two main thyroid hormones are triiodothyronine (T3) and thyroxine (T4), both of which help control the speed at which the body uses energy.

When the thyroid functions properly, it helps maintain a balance between burning and storing energy. However, hypothyroidism (an underactive thyroid) slows metabolism, making it easier to gain weight and harder to lose it. Conversely, hyperthyroidism (an overactive thyroid) speeds up metabolism, potentially leading to unintentional weight loss.

Hypothyroidism and Weight Gain

In cases of hypothyroidism, the thyroid gland produces insufficient amounts of T3 and T4, which can lead to a slower metabolism. Symptoms of hypothyroidism often include:

- Weight gain
- Fatigue
- Cold intolerance
- Hair thinning
- Depression

One study published in *The Lancet Diabetes & Endocrinology* (Chaker et al., 2017) found that hypothyroidism is associated with increased weight gain and difficulty in weight loss, even with calorie restriction and exercise.

Ways to Improve Thyroid Function Naturally

While medication is often required to manage clinical hypothyroidism, certain lifestyle changes and nutrients can support thyroid function and optimize metabolism naturally:

- **Iodine:** Iodine is essential for thyroid hormone production. Foods like seaweed, fish, dairy, and iodized salt are rich sources of iodine.
- **Selenium:** Selenium helps convert T4 into the active form T3. Brazil nuts, sunflower seeds, and tuna are excellent sources of selenium. Research published in the *Journal of Clinical Endocrinology & Metabolism* (Ventura et al., 2017) suggests that selenium supplementation may improve thyroid function in patients with autoimmune thyroiditis.
- **Zinc:** Zinc is another mineral crucial for thyroid function. Foods rich in zinc include oysters, beef, and pumpkin seeds. A 2013 study published in the *Journal of the American College of Nutri-*

tion found that zinc supplementation improved thyroid function in women with mild hypothyroidism.

▸ **Vitamin D:** Vitamin D deficiency is linked to thyroid dysfunction. Spending time in the sun or consuming foods like fortified dairy and fatty fish can boost vitamin D levels.

▸ **Reduce stress:** Chronic stress can affect thyroid function by disrupting the hypothalamic-pituitary-thyroid (HPT) axis. Practicing relaxation techniques like yoga, meditation, and deep breathing may help reduce stress and improve thyroid function.

Insulin: The Fat-Storing Hormone

Insulin is a hormone produced by the pancreas that helps regulate blood sugar levels. When you eat carbohydrates, insulin is released to shuttle glucose (sugar) into cells for energy or storage. However, when insulin levels are chronically elevated—often due to a high-carb diet or insulin resistance—excess glucose is stored as fat.

People with insulin resistance tend to store fat more easily, particularly around the abdomen, which increases the risk of metabolic disorders like type 2 diabetes and cardiovascular disease. Insulin resistance also makes it harder to burn fat for energy, which can stall weight loss efforts.

To improve insulin sensitivity and promote fat loss:

▸ **Adopt a low-carb diet:** Reducing carbohydrate intake can lower insulin levels and promote fat burning.

▸ **Exercise regularly:** Physical activity, particularly strength training, can increase insulin sensitivity and help the body use glucose more effectively.

▶ **Increase fiber intake:** High-fiber foods like vegetables, legumes, and whole grains slow the release of glucose into the bloodstream, reducing insulin spikes.

Leptin: The Hunger Regulator

Leptin is a hormone produced by fat cells that signals to the brain when the body has enough energy stored. Essentially, leptin tells your brain when to stop eating. However, in people with obesity, leptin resistance can occur, meaning the brain no longer responds to leptin signals properly. This can lead to overeating and difficulty losing weight.

One way to improve leptin sensitivity is by getting enough sleep. Studies have shown that sleep deprivation can reduce leptin levels and increase hunger, making it harder to maintain a healthy weight. Additionally, consuming a diet rich in omega-3 fatty acids (found in fatty fish, walnuts, and flaxseeds) may help improve leptin sensitivity and reduce inflammation.

Cortisol: The Stress Hormone and Its Impact on Fat Storage

Cortisol is a hormone produced by the adrenal glands in response to stress. It plays an important role in various bodily functions, including metabolism, immune response, and blood sugar regulation. However, chronic stress and elevated cortisol levels can lead to weight gain, especially around the midsection, due to increased fat storage.

How Cortisol Contributes to Weight Gain

Cortisol promotes the breakdown of muscle for energy and increases blood sugar levels to prepare the body for a "fight or flight" response. This rise in blood sugar stimulates insulin release, which, over time, can lead to insulin resistance and fat storage. Elevated cortisol also increases cravings for high-calorie, sugary, and fatty foods, further contributing to weight gain.

Ways to Improve Cortisol Levels Naturally

Lowering cortisol levels can significantly reduce the tendency to store fat and promote weight loss. Natural ways to balance cortisol include:

- ▸ **Manage stress:** Practicing stress-reducing techniques like mindfulness, meditation, and yoga can help lower cortisol levels. A study published in *Health Psychology* (Epel et al., 2004) showed that individuals who practiced mindfulness had lower cortisol levels and reduced belly fat.

- ▸ **Adequate sleep:** Sleep deprivation increases cortisol production. Prioritize 7-9 hours of sleep per night to keep cortisol in check and improve overall health.

- ▸ **Exercise:** Moderate-intensity exercise, like walking or yoga, can reduce cortisol levels. However, excessive high-intensity exercise can increase cortisol, so balance is key.

- ▸ **Ashwagandha:** This adaptogenic herb has been shown in clinical trials to reduce cortisol levels and improve stress resilience. A study published in the *Indian Journal of Psychological Medicine* (Chandrasekhar et al., 2012) found that Ashwagandha supplementation significantly lowered cortisol in chronically stressed adults.

Conclusion

Metabolic rate and hormonal balance are critical determinants of fat storage, weight loss, and overall health. Hormones like thyroid hormone, insulin, leptin, and cortisol all play vital roles in regulating metabolism and body fat. By optimizing thyroid function through proper nutrition, reducing stress to control cortisol, and improving insulin and leptin sensitivity through lifestyle changes, individuals can take control of their metabolism and achieve sustainable weight loss. Understanding the intricate relationship between hormones and fat storage is key to long-term health and successful weight management.

"*To keep the body in good health is a duty... otherwise we shall not be able to keep our mind strong and clear.*"

– BUDDHA

CHAPTER 4

Nutritional Counseling
Creating Tailored Diets for Lasting Weight Loss and Health

Introduction

Nutritional counseling is a powerful tool for individuals aiming to lose weight, manage chronic conditions, and improve overall health. Unlike fad diets that promise rapid results but often lead to yo-yo dieting, nutritional counseling emphasizes personalized diets that focus on caloric deficits, macronutrient balance, and long-term lifestyle changes. The goal is to create a sustainable, healthy way of eating that promotes weight loss, reduces cholesterol, stabilizes blood sugar levels, and supports muscle retention through protein-rich foods.

In this chapter, we will explore how nutritional counseling can help individuals achieve these goals, examining the role of caloric balance, macronutrients, and providing sample meals and recipes designed to support long-term health.

The Importance of Caloric Deficits for Weight Loss

Weight loss fundamentally comes down to creating a caloric deficit, where you consume fewer calories than your body needs to maintain its current weight. According to the National Institutes of Health (NIH), a caloric deficit of about 500-1,000 calories per day can lead to a healthy weight loss of 1-2 pounds per week. While this may sound simple, creating a sustainable caloric deficit requires careful consideration of nutrient density and macronutrient balance to ensure the body is still receiving the vitamins, minerals, and energy it needs to function optimally.

Macronutrient Balance for Optimal Health and Weight Loss

Macronutrients—carbohydrates, proteins, and fats—play distinct roles in how the body processes energy, builds muscle, and stores fat. The right balance of macronutrients can enhance weight loss, improve satiety, and support metabolic health.

▶ **Protein:** Protein is essential for muscle maintenance and repair, especially during weight loss. High-protein diets increase satiety and help reduce overall calorie intake. Research published in the *American Journal of Clinical Nutrition* found that diets high in protein (about 25-30% of total caloric intake) are associated with greater weight loss and fat loss, compared to lower-protein diets. Additionally, protein is critical for preserving lean muscle mass while in a caloric deficit.

▶ **Recommended intake:** 20-30% of total daily calories

▶ **Sources:** Chicken, turkey, lean beef, tofu, legumes, fish, eggs, and Greek yogurt.

▶ **Carbohydrates:** Carbohydrates are the body's primary energy source, but not all carbs are created equal. Low-carbohydrate diets, particularly those focusing on complex carbohydrates and fiber-rich foods, can be effective for weight loss and blood sugar control. Refined carbohydrates, such as white bread, sugary snacks, and soda, spike insulin levels and can promote fat storage. Studies suggest that low-carb diets (particularly those with fewer than 130 grams of carbs per day) can be beneficial for individuals with insulin resistance or type 2 diabetes by improving blood sugar control and promoting fat loss.

▸ **Recommended intake:** 20-50% of total daily calories, depending on individual needs.

▸ **Sources:** Whole grains, sweet potatoes, leafy green vegetables, berries, legumes, and oats.

▸ **Fats:** Healthy fats are crucial for hormone production, brain function, and the absorption of fat-soluble vitamins. Unsaturated fats, found in foods like olive oil, nuts, seeds, and avocados, can improve cholesterol levels and promote heart health, while trans fats and excessive saturated fats contribute to weight gain and elevated cholesterol levels. A balanced approach to fat intake, where healthy fats make up around 20-35% of total daily calories, supports long-term health and satiety.

▸ **Recommended intake:** 20-35% of total daily calories.

▸ **Sources:** Olive oil, nuts, seeds, fatty fish (like salmon), avocado, and flaxseeds.

Tailored Diets for Specific Health Goals

Effective nutritional counseling goes beyond weight loss and addresses specific health conditions such as high cholesterol, diabetes, and muscle retention. By tailoring macronutrient intake and food choices, a personalized diet can help individuals achieve their health goals in a sustainable way.

Low Cholesterol Diets

For individuals with high cholesterol, focusing on heart-healthy foods is essential. Nutritional counseling will often incorporate:

- **Soluble fiber:** This type of fiber helps reduce LDL ("bad") cholesterol levels. Foods like oats, beans, lentils, apples, and flaxseeds are excellent sources of soluble fiber.
- **Healthy fats:** Replacing saturated fats with unsaturated fats from sources like olive oil, nuts, and fatty fish can improve cholesterol levels.
- **Plant sterols:** Found in fortified foods, plant sterols help block cholesterol absorption in the intestines.

Sample Day of Eating:

- **Breakfast:** Oatmeal topped with chia seeds, flaxseeds, and fresh berries.
- **Lunch:** Quinoa salad with mixed greens, chickpeas, avocado, and a lemon-olive oil dressing.
- **Dinner:** Grilled salmon with a side of roasted Brussels sprouts and sweet potatoes.
- **Snack:** A handful of almonds or walnuts.

Low Sugar, Low-Carbohydrate Diets

For those struggling with insulin resistance or type 2 diabetes, controlling blood sugar levels through diet is paramount. Nutritional counseling will emphasize:

- **Low-glycemic foods:** Foods that have a low impact on blood sugar, such as leafy greens, non-starchy vegetables, and legumes.

▶ **Healthy fats and proteins:** Including more protein and healthy fats helps stabilize blood sugar and promote satiety.

▶ **Limiting refined sugars and processed carbs:** Cutting out sugary drinks, candy, and white bread reduces blood sugar spikes.

Sample Day of Eating:

▶ **Breakfast:** Scrambled eggs with spinach and avocado.

▶ **Lunch:** Grilled chicken salad with mixed greens, olive oil, and balsamic vinegar.

▶ **Dinner:** Baked cod with sautéed kale and cauliflower mash.

▶ **Snack:** Greek yogurt with a few sliced almonds and cinnamon.

High-Protein, Muscle-Supporting Diets

For individuals focused on maintaining or building lean muscle while losing fat, a high-protein diet is crucial. Nutritional counseling for muscle retention will focus on:

▶ **Adequate protein intake:** Ensuring protein intake remains high enough to support muscle synthesis, particularly for those engaging in strength training.

▶ **Balanced meals:** Including protein at every meal to promote muscle repair and recovery.

▶ **Complex carbohydrates:** Supporting workouts with nutrient-dense carbs like brown rice, quinoa, and sweet potatoes to fuel exercise.

Sample Day of Eating:

▶ **Breakfast:** Greek yogurt parfait with mixed berries, chia seeds, and a drizzle of honey.

▶ **Lunch:** Grilled turkey burger on a whole grain bun with a side of roasted vegetables.

> **Dinner:** Grilled chicken breast with quinoa, steamed broccoli, and a sprinkle of feta cheese.

> **Snack:** Cottage cheese with sliced cucumber and cherry tomatoes.

Long-Term Lifestyle Changes for Sustainable Health

Sustainable weight loss and health improvements require more than just short-term changes to diet. Nutritional counseling emphasizes long-term lifestyle changes that ensure individuals can maintain their progress over time.

> **Meal planning:** Preparing meals in advance helps prevent impulsive eating and makes it easier to stick to a healthy diet. Individuals are encouraged to plan meals for the week, including plenty of vegetables, lean proteins, and healthy fats.

> **Portion control:** While eating nutrient-dense foods is important, portion control is key to maintaining a caloric deficit. Using smaller plates, measuring portions, and being mindful of serving sizes can help prevent overeating.

> **Mindful eating:** Paying attention to hunger and fullness cues, eating slowly, and avoiding distractions while eating are important components of mindful eating. Research has shown that people who practice mindful eating are more likely to lose weight and maintain it.

> **Physical activity:** While diet is crucial for weight loss, combining it with regular exercise can enhance results. Strength training helps preserve muscle mass during weight loss, while cardio exercises support fat burning and heart health.

Sample Recipes for Healthy Eating

Breakfast: Spinach and Feta Omelet

Ingredients:

- 2 eggs
- 1 cup fresh spinach
- 1 oz feta cheese
- 1 tsp olive oil
- Salt and pepper to taste

Instructions:

1. Heat olive oil in a skillet over medium heat. Add spinach and cook until wilted.
2. In a bowl, whisk eggs, then pour over spinach.
3. Cook until eggs are almost set, then sprinkle feta cheese on top.
4. Fold the omelet in half, cook for an additional minute, then serve.

Lunch: Grilled Chicken and Quinoa Salad

Ingredients:

- 4 oz grilled chicken breast
- ½ cup cooked quinoa
- 1 cup mixed greens
- 1 tbsp olive oil
- 1 tbsp balsamic vinegar
- Salt and pepper to taste

Instructions:

1. In a bowl, combine mixed greens, quinoa, and grilled chicken.
2. Drizzle with olive oil and balsamic vinegar, season with salt and pepper, and toss to combine.

25

Dinner: Baked Salmon with Sweet Potatoes and Asparagus

Ingredients:

- ▶ 6 oz salmon fillet
- ▶ 1 medium sweet potato, sliced
- ▶ 1 cup asparagus spears
- ▶ 1 tsp olive oil
- ▶ Salt, pepper, and garlic powder to taste

"Your body will be around a lot longer than that expensive handbag. Invest in yourself."

– UNKNOWN

CHAPTER 5

Behavioral Therapy

Cognitive-Behavioral Approaches for Changing Eating Habits and Emotional Eating

Introduction

Changing eating habits and maintaining a weight loss plan is not just about understanding what to eat; it's also about changing the psychological patterns that often lead to overeating or poor food choices. Cognitive-Behavioral Therapy (CBT) is one of the most effective tools used in behavioral therapy to address challenges like emotional eating, stress eating, and lapses in diet adherence. By focusing on the connection between thoughts, emotions, and behaviors, CBT helps individuals gain control over their relationship with food, create healthier eating habits, and sustain long-term weight loss.

This chapter will explore how behavioral therapy, particularly CBT, can be applied to weight management, emotional eating, and the formation of long-term healthy eating habits. We'll also discuss the latest research supporting the effectiveness of these approaches and how compassionate, non-judgmental strategies can make a significant difference in promoting lasting change.

Understanding the Cognitive-Behavioral Approach

Cognitive-Behavioral Therapy is based on the idea that our thoughts (cognitions) influence our feelings and behaviors. In the context of weight loss and eating habits, negative or distorted thinking patterns often lead to behaviors like overeating or making unhealthy food choices. By identifying these thought patterns and replacing them with more realistic, constructive thoughts, individuals can break the cycle of emotional eating and develop healthier behaviors.

CBT focuses on three main areas:

▸ **Identifying problematic thoughts:** These may include beliefs like "I've ruined my diet, so I may as well eat whatever I want" or "I'm a failure because I can't stick to my plan."

▸ **Challenging and reframing these thoughts:** Instead of letting negative thoughts dictate behavior, CBT encourages questioning these beliefs and reframing them. For example, replacing "I've ruined my diet" with "One slip-up doesn't mean I've failed. I can get back on track."

▸ **Developing new coping strategies:** This involves finding healthier ways to cope with emotions like stress, sadness, or boredom, which often trigger emotional eating.

Emotional Eating: A Common Barrier to Weight Loss

One of the most significant challenges people face in maintaining a healthy weight is emotional eating. Emotional eating refers to eating in response to feelings rather than hunger. According to a study published in *Appetite* (van Strien et al., 2013), emotional eaters are more likely to consume high-calorie, sugary foods when experiencing negative emotions like stress, anxiety, loneliness, or boredom. These behaviors often lead to weight gain, frustration, and feelings of guilt, creating a vicious cycle of unhealthy eating.

Recognizing Triggers

A core component of CBT is helping individuals recognize their emotional eating triggers. These may include:

- **Stress:** High-stress situations, whether related to work, family, or finances, often lead people to seek comfort in food.
- **Boredom:** Eating out of boredom or to fill time is a common issue, particularly when food becomes a form of entertainment or distraction.
- **Sadness or Loneliness:** Emotional voids are often temporarily filled by eating, especially foods associated with comfort or pleasure.
- **Social Influences:** Eating can become a coping mechanism in social situations where food plays a central role, such as parties, gatherings, or celebrations.

By becoming aware of these triggers, individuals can begin to anticipate and prepare for situations where they might be tempted to eat emotionally, rather than react impulsively.

Developing Alternative Coping Mechanisms

Once emotional eating triggers are identified, CBT focuses on developing alternative coping strategies that don't involve food. Some effective techniques include:

- **Mindful breathing:** Learning to take deep breaths and center oneself during stressful moments can reduce the immediate urge to turn to food.
- **Journaling:** Writing down thoughts and emotions can help individuals process their feelings without eating.

> **Physical activity:** Going for a walk, practicing yoga, or engaging in another form of physical activity can relieve stress and provide a positive outlet for emotions.

> **Engaging in a hobby:** Redirecting focus to a hobby or creative activity can take attention away from the desire to eat and provide a sense of fulfillment.

Changing Eating Habits Through Cognitive Restructuring

Another key aspect of behavioral therapy is cognitive restructuring, which involves identifying and challenging unhealthy thought patterns related to eating and self-image. Many people struggling with weight loss often hold all-or-nothing thinking, where they believe that any deviation from their diet is a complete failure. This mindset can lead to binge eating or giving up on weight loss goals entirely after minor slip-ups.

For example, after eating a high-calorie dessert, someone might think, "I've failed today. I'll never lose weight." CBT helps individuals change these thoughts to something more balanced, such as, "I had a treat, but that doesn't mean I've ruined my progress. I can make healthier choices the rest of the day."

A study published in *Obesity Research* (Wadden et al., 2005) found that participants who underwent CBT for weight loss were more successful in maintaining weight loss compared to those who followed traditional diet and exercise plans. The CBT group was better equipped to handle setbacks, leading to more consistent long-term results.

Increasing Adherence to Weight Loss Plans

One of the biggest challenges in weight loss is maintaining motivation and adherence to a plan over the long term. Behavioral therapy addresses this by helping individuals set realistic goals and focus on incremental progress rather than perfection.

Setting Realistic and Achievable Goals

Setting unrealistic or overly ambitious goals often leads to frustration and early abandonment of weight loss efforts. Behavioral therapy encourages individuals to set small, attainable goals that build confidence and create a sense of accomplishment. For example, instead of aiming to lose 20 pounds in a month, a more realistic goal would be to aim for 1-2 pounds of weight loss per week, which is more sustainable and easier to achieve.

Fostering Self-Compassion and Positive Reinforcement

CBT also promotes self-compassion, encouraging individuals to be kind to themselves when they experience setbacks. Research published in *Obesity* (Lillis et al., 2016) shows that individuals who practice self-compassion are more likely to stay motivated and adhere to their weight loss goals. Instead of focusing on failures, CBT teaches individuals to celebrate small victories, such as sticking to a meal plan for the day or incorporating more fruits and vegetables into meals.

Using positive reinforcement, such as rewarding oneself for reaching a weekly goal (e.g., with a non-food treat like a new book or an activity you enjoy), can also strengthen adherence and build momentum over time.

Mindfulness and Behavioral Therapy

In recent years, integrating mindfulness techniques with CBT has gained attention for its role in reducing emotional eating and promoting healthy eating behaviors. Mindful eating involves paying full attention to the act of eating, including the taste, texture, and smell of food, as well as recognizing hunger and fullness cues.

A study in *Eating Behaviors* (Tapper et al., 2009) found that participants who practiced mindful eating alongside CBT interventions were more successful in reducing binge eating episodes and improving their relationship with food. Mindfulness helps individuals eat more slowly, enjoy their food, and recognize when they are full, leading to fewer overeating episodes.

Some key mindfulness strategies include:

> ▸ **Slowing down:** Taking time to chew food thoroughly and savor each bite can increase satisfaction and reduce the likelihood of overeating.

> ▸ **Listening to hunger cues:** Learning to distinguish between physical hunger and emotional cravings can help prevent unnecessary eating.

> ▸ **Eliminating distractions:** Avoiding distractions like TV or smartphones during meals helps individuals focus on the experience of eating and recognize when they're full.

Conclusion

Behavioral therapy, particularly through the use of Cognitive-Behavioral Therapy, is a highly effective tool for changing eating habits, addressing emotional eating, and increasing adherence to weight loss plans. By focusing on the connection between thoughts, emotions, and behaviors, CBT provides individuals with the skills needed to overcome negative patterns and develop healthier relationships with food.

Through recognizing triggers, developing alternative coping mechanisms, practicing mindfulness, and fostering self-compassion, behavioral therapy empowers individuals to take control of their eating habits and achieve lasting success in weight management. Ultimately, combining these psychological approaches with a balanced diet and regular physical activity creates a holistic, sustainable strategy for long-term health and well-being.

"Health is not about the weight you lose but about the life you gain."

– DR. JOSH AXE

CHAPTER 6

Exercise Prescription

Structured Programs for Fat Loss, Muscle Preservation, and Metabolic Health

Introduction

Exercise is a critical component of any effective weight loss program, especially when it comes to fat loss, muscle preservation, and metabolic health. A well-structured exercise program not only burns calories but also improves cardiovascular health, strengthens muscles, and enhances metabolic function. For individuals dealing with conditions like diabetes or obesity, exercise becomes even more essential, as it helps manage blood sugar levels and reduce excess weight, mitigating risks associated with these conditions.

In this chapter, we will explore different types of exercise programs, including those focused on fat loss, muscle building, and endurance. We'll also discuss how structured exercise programs can be tailored to individuals with diabetes or obesity, providing examples of effective routines designed to meet their specific needs.

The Role of Exercise in Fat Loss

Exercise for fat loss revolves around creating a caloric deficit, where the body burns more calories than it consumes. While diet is the primary driver of fat loss, exercise enhances the process by increasing the number of calories burned daily. However, not all forms of exercise are equally effective for fat loss. Combining aerobic exercises, such as running or cycling, with strength training creates a balanced program that promotes fat loss while preserving lean muscle mass.

Example Fat Loss Exercise Program

A well-rounded fat loss program includes both cardiovascular (aerobic) exercises and resistance training to maximize calorie burn and muscle preservation.

Sample Program:

Day 1: Full-Body Strength Training (45 minutes)

- Squats: 3 sets of 12 reps
- Push-ups: 3 sets of 10-12 reps
- Bent-over rows: 3 sets of 12 reps
- Lunges: 3 sets of 12 reps (each leg)
- Plank: 3 sets, hold for 30-60 seconds

Day 2: High-Intensity Interval Training (HIIT) (30 minutes)

- Warm-up: 5 minutes of light jogging or brisk walking
- 30 seconds of sprinting followed by 90 seconds of walking or slow jogging (repeat 8 times)
- Cool down: 5 minutes of light walking

Day 3: Rest or Light Activity (e.g., walking or yoga)

Day 4: Upper Body Strength Training (45 minutes)

- Bench press or dumbbell chest press: 3 sets of 10 reps
- Shoulder press: 3 sets of 10 reps
- Bicep curls: 3 sets of 12 reps

- Tricep dips: 3 sets of 12 reps
- Bicycle crunches: 3 sets of 20 reps

Day 5: Steady-State Cardio (45 minutes)

- Moderate-intensity cycling, jogging, or swimming

Day 6: Lower Body Strength Training (45 minutes)

- Deadlifts: 3 sets of 10 reps
- Step-ups: 3 sets of 12 reps (each leg)
- Leg press: 3 sets of 10 reps
- Calf raises: 3 sets of 15 reps
- Side plank: 3 sets, hold for 30 seconds each side

Day 7: Rest or Light Activity

This program combines strength training to preserve muscle with cardio and HIIT to maximize calorie burn, promoting fat loss while maintaining lean mass.

Exercise for Muscle Building

Building muscle is a key goal for many individuals, particularly those looking to improve their body composition. Strength training is the cornerstone of muscle building, as it stimulates muscle hypertrophy through progressive overload, where muscles are gradually exposed to increased resistance over time. Incorporating a variety of compound and isolation exercises ensures that all major muscle groups are targeted.

Example Muscle Building Program

Sample Program:

- ▶ Day 1: Push Day (Chest, Shoulders, Triceps)
- ▶ Bench press: 4 sets of 8-10 reps
- ▶ Overhead shoulder press: 4 sets of 8-10 reps
- ▶ Incline dumbbell press: 3 sets of 8-10 reps
- ▶ Tricep dips: 3 sets of 12 reps
- ▶ Side lateral raises: 3 sets of 12-15 reps
- ▶ Day 2: Pull Day (Back, Biceps)
- ▶ Deadlifts: 4 sets of 6-8 reps
- ▶ Pull-ups or lat pulldowns: 4 sets of 8-10 reps
- ▶ Bent-over rows: 3 sets of 8-10 reps
- ▶ Dumbbell bicep curls: 3 sets of 10-12 reps
- ▶ Face pulls: 3 sets of 12-15 reps
- ▶ Day 3: Rest or Active Recovery
- ▶ Day 4: Leg Day (Quads, Hamstrings, Glutes)
- ▶ Squats: 4 sets of 8-10 reps
- ▶ Leg press: 4 sets of 10 reps
- ▶ Romanian deadlifts: 3 sets of 8-10 reps
- ▶ Walking lunges: 3 sets of 12 reps (each leg)
- ▶ Calf raises: 3 sets of 15-20 reps
- ▶ Day 5: Upper Body Isolation (Arms, Shoulders)
- ▶ Barbell curls: 3 sets of 8-10 reps
- ▶ Tricep pushdowns: 3 sets of 10-12 reps
- ▶ Arnold press: 3 sets of 8-10 reps
- ▶ Shrugs: 3 sets of 12 reps
- ▶ Hammer curls: 3 sets of 10-12 reps

Muscle building programs are characterized by progressive overload—gradually increasing weight or resistance over time to continuously challenge muscles and promote growth. Adequate rest between sets and workout days is essential to allow for muscle recovery and repair.

Exercise for Increasing Endurance

Endurance training focuses on improving the body's ability to sustain prolonged physical activity. For those seeking to increase cardiovascular endurance, activities like long-distance running, cycling, or swimming are effective. These activities improve the heart's ability to pump blood efficiently and increase lung capacity.

Example Endurance Program

Sample Program:

- Day 1: Long Run (60 minutes)
- Run at a moderate, steady pace for 60 minutes, aiming to maintain a consistent heart rate in the aerobic zone (about 60-70% of max heart rate).
- Day 2: Interval Training (30 minutes)
- Warm-up: 5 minutes of light jogging
- 1-minute sprint, followed by 2 minutes of walking or jogging (repeat 10 times)
- Cool down: 5 minutes of light jogging or walking
- Day 3: Cross-Training (e.g., cycling or swimming) (45-60 minutes)
- Day 4: Rest or Light Activity (e.g., yoga or walking)
- Day 5: Tempo Run (40 minutes)
- Run at a challenging but sustainable pace for 40 minutes, targeting 80% of your max heart rate.
- Day 6: Strength Training (Full Body) (45 minutes)
- Day 7: Rest or Light Activity

By alternating between steady-state cardio, interval training, and tempo runs, this program enhances both aerobic and anaerobic endurance, improving stamina over time.

Exercise for People with Diabetes

For individuals with diabetes, structured exercise programs can help regulate blood sugar levels, improve insulin sensitivity, and promote weight loss. According to the American Diabetes Association (ADA), both aerobic and resistance training are recommended for diabetes management. Exercise improves the body's ability to use insulin, making it easier to control blood sugar levels.

Example Exercise Program for Diabetes

Sample Program:

- ▶ Day 1: Aerobic Exercise (30-45 minutes)
- ▶ Brisk walking, cycling, or swimming at a moderate intensity.
- ▶ Day 2: Strength Training (Full Body) (45 minutes)
- ▶ Bodyweight exercises like squats, lunges, push-ups, and resistance band exercises.
- ▶ Dumbbell or machine exercises targeting major muscle groups.
- ▶ Day 3: Rest or Light Activity
- ▶ Day 4: Interval Training (30 minutes)
- ▶ 30 seconds of high-intensity exercise (e.g., sprinting or cycling), followed by 2 minutes of rest or low-intensity exercise (e.g., walking or slow cycling). Repeat 8-10 times.
- ▶ Day 5: Strength Training (Full Body) (45 minutes)
- ▶ Day 6: Aerobic Exercise (45-60 minutes)
- ▶ Walking, cycling, or swimming at a moderate pace.
- ▶ Day 7: Rest or Light Activity

This program combines aerobic activity to improve cardiovascular health and insulin sensitivity with strength training to build muscle mass, which further enhances glucose regulation.

Exercise for People Who Are Overweight

For individuals who are overweight, exercise programs should be designed to reduce excess weight without placing undue stress on the joints. Low-impact exercises like swimming, cycling, and walking are often recommended to minimize the risk of injury while promoting fat loss and muscle gain.

Example Exercise Program for Overweight Individuals

Sample Programs:

Day 1: Low-Impact Aerobic

Low-impact exercises are ideal for individuals who are overweight, have joint issues, or are new to exercising, as they minimize stress on the body while promoting fat loss, cardiovascular health, and muscle strength. Here are some effective examples:

1. **Walking:** A simple and accessible exercise that can be done almost anywhere. Walking improves cardiovascular endurance, burns calories, and is gentle on the joints.
2. **Swimming:** An excellent full-body workout that increases heart rate without putting pressure on joints. The water provides resistance, making it great for toning muscles while being low-impact.
3. **Cycling:** Whether on a stationary bike or a regular bicycle, cycling is a great way to improve cardiovascular fitness and strengthen leg muscles while being easy on the knees and hips.

4. **Elliptical Training:** Using an elliptical machine provides a full-body workout with minimal impact on the joints. It mimics walking or running movements without the jarring effect of pounding the pavement.

5. **Yoga:** Yoga combines flexibility, balance, and strength training while being gentle on the body. It also helps improve mental well-being and reduces stress.

6. **Water Aerobics:** Similar to swimming, this activity offers a full-body workout with resistance from the water, making it ideal for burning calories and building strength without joint strain.

These exercises promote overall fitness while minimizing injury risk, making them suitable for long-term, sustainable weight loss.

"A healthy outside starts from the inside."

– ROBERT URICH

CHAPTER 7

Gut Health & Microbiome

The Influence of Gut Bacteria on Weight Management

Introduction

In recent years, gut health has emerged as a key factor in overall well-being, with research showing that the gut microbiome—the trillions of microorganisms living in our digestive system—plays a crucial role in weight management, metabolic health, and even mood regulation. The balance and diversity of gut bacteria have been linked to how efficiently we process food, store fat, and regulate hormones related to hunger and satiety.

In this chapter, we will explore the connection between the gut microbiome and weight management, the role of probiotics, prebiotics, and fiber in fat loss, and how certain digestive disorders can impact nutrient absorption. We'll also provide examples of fiber-rich foods that support gut health and weight management.

The Gut Microbiome and Weight Management

The gut microbiome is composed of a diverse array of bacteria, fungi, and viruses that live in our intestines. These microorganisms help with the digestion of food, the production of essential vitamins, and the regulation of our immune system. Recent research has shown that the gut microbiome is also deeply intertwined with our metabolism and weight management.

Studies have found that gut bacteria can influence how the body stores fat and how it balances blood sugar. For example, people with obesity tend to have a different composition of gut bacteria compared to those with healthy body weight. Specifically, they tend to have fewer Bacteroidetes and more Firmicutes, a bacterial ratio associated with higher fat storage. The exact mechanisms behind this imbalance are still being explored, but it's clear that the gut microbiome plays a role in energy extraction from food and fat storage.

Moreover, gut bacteria produce short-chain fatty acids (SCFAs) from fiber fermentation. These SCFAs, like butyrate, propionate, and acetate, have been shown to influence appetite regulation by communicating with hunger hormones like ghrelin and leptin, and they can also reduce inflammation, which is associated with obesity and metabolic disorders.

Probiotics, Prebiotics, and Fat Loss

Improving the balance of gut bacteria through diet and supplements can positively affect weight management. Probiotics and prebiotics are two essential elements in this process.

Probiotics

Probiotics are live microorganisms, usually specific strains of bacteria or yeast, that can be consumed through supplements or fermented foods. They help maintain or restore the balance of the gut microbiome by increasing the number of beneficial bacteria.

Certain probiotic strains have been associated with fat loss and better metabolic health. For example:

- **Lactobacillus gasseri:** This strain has been shown to reduce abdominal fat in several studies. A study published in the journal *European Journal of Clinical Nutrition* found that individuals who consumed Lactobacillus gasseri daily for 12 weeks saw significant reductions in belly fat.
- **Bifidobacterium animalis:** This strain has been linked to reduced body fat and improved digestion in several studies.

Fermented foods that are rich in probiotics include:

- Yogurt (with live cultures)
- Kefir
- Sauerkraut
- Kimchi
- Miso
- Tempeh

These foods not only introduce beneficial bacteria to the gut but also help to enhance digestion and the absorption of nutrients, which can contribute to better weight management.

Prebiotics

Prebiotics are non-digestible fibers that serve as food for beneficial gut bacteria. These fibers pass through the digestive system without being broken down and provide sustenance for the gut microbiota. Feeding the gut bacteria with prebiotics helps maintain a healthy and diverse microbial environment, which is crucial for weight management and overall health.

Foods rich in prebiotics include:

- Garlic
- Onions
- Leeks

- Asparagus
- Bananas
- Jerusalem artichokes
- Chicory root

By nourishing beneficial bacteria, prebiotics promote a healthy gut environment that can enhance fat metabolism and reduce inflammation.

The Role of Fiber in Weight Loss

Fiber is a type of carbohydrate that the body cannot digest, but it plays an important role in supporting gut health and weight management. There are two types of dietary fiber: soluble and insoluble.

- Soluble fiber dissolves in water and forms a gel-like substance in the gut. This helps slow down digestion, promote satiety, and reduce calorie intake. Soluble fiber also helps regulate blood sugar levels by slowing the absorption of sugar, making it particularly beneficial for individuals with diabetes or insulin resistance.
- Insoluble fiber adds bulk to the stool and helps maintain regular bowel movements. While it doesn't directly contribute to fat loss, it promotes a healthy digestive system by preventing constipation and supporting the growth of beneficial gut bacteria.

Fiber also plays a significant role in promoting the production of SCFAs, which, as previously mentioned, help regulate appetite and reduce inflammation. Additionally, high-fiber foods tend to be lower in calories, making them ideal for those looking to create a caloric deficit.

Examples of Fiber-Rich Foods

Foods high in fiber that support both gut health and weight loss include:

- **Oats:** Rich in beta-glucan, a type of soluble fiber that promotes satiety and reduces cholesterol levels.
- **Chia seeds:** Packed with fiber, chia seeds expand in the stomach, promoting fullness and reducing overall calorie intake.
- **Legumes:** Beans, lentils, and chickpeas are excellent sources of both soluble and insoluble fiber.
- **Berries:** Low in sugar but high in fiber, berries like raspberries, blackberries, and strawberries are perfect for weight loss diets.
- **Whole grains:** Foods like quinoa, brown rice, and barley are high in insoluble fiber, which supports digestion.
- **Vegetables:** Non-starchy vegetables like broccoli, Brussels sprouts, and spinach provide fiber without adding many calories.

Digestive Disorders and Absorption

When the gut is unhealthy, it can impact nutrient absorption and digestion, which in turn affects weight management. Digestive disorders like Irritable Bowel Syndrome (IBS), Crohn's disease, and celiac disease can alter the balance of the gut microbiome and interfere with the absorption of vital nutrients, leading to malnutrition or unintended weight changes.

For example:

- Celiac disease damages the lining of the small intestine, leading to malabsorption of nutrients like iron and calcium. This can result in weight loss and nutrient deficiencies.

▶ Crohn's disease, a type of inflammatory bowel disease (IBD), can cause inflammation in the digestive tract, leading to diarrhea, malnutrition, and weight fluctuations.

▶ IBS can lead to symptoms like bloating, constipation, and diarrhea, which affect how efficiently the body processes food and absorbs nutrients.

In individuals with digestive disorders, improving gut health through a low-FODMAP diet (which reduces certain fermentable carbohydrates) or incorporating probiotics and prebiotics can alleviate symptoms and improve nutrient absorption.

Improving Gut Health for Weight Loss

There are several strategies to improve gut health and support weight loss:

1. **Incorporate probiotics and prebiotics:** Eating fermented foods and high-fiber, prebiotic-rich foods can increase beneficial bacteria and improve digestion.

2. **Increase fiber intake:** Eating plenty of fruits, vegetables, legumes, and whole grains supports gut health and promotes fat loss.

3. **Stay hydrated:** Water helps fiber move through the digestive system and keeps the gut functioning properly.

4. **Limit processed foods and sugar:** Highly processed foods and added sugars can negatively impact the gut microbiome and contribute to weight gain.

5. **Exercise regularly:** Physical activity has been shown to increase the diversity of gut bacteria and improve overall gut health.

Conclusion

The connection between gut health and weight management is becoming increasingly clear. The gut microbiome plays a vital role in how we process food, store fat, and regulate appetite. By incorporating probiotics, prebiotics, and fiber into our diets, we can improve gut health, support fat loss, and enhance overall well-being. Additionally, understanding how digestive disorders affect nutrient absorption allows individuals to tailor their diets to improve both gut health and metabolic function.

By making these changes, individuals can harness the power of the gut microbiome to achieve better health outcomes and sustainable weight loss.

"It is health that is real wealth and not pieces of gold and silver."

– MAHATMA GANDHI

CHAPTER 8

Medical Conditions & Weight

Addressing Challenges in Weight Loss with Hypothyroidism, PCOS, and Diabetes

Introduction

Losing weight is challenging for most people, but certain medical conditions can make weight loss efforts even more difficult. Conditions such as hypothyroidism, Polycystic Ovary Syndrome (PCOS), and diabetes not only complicate the body's ability to shed excess fat but also require specialized treatment to avoid negative health outcomes. Without proper medical supervision, individuals with these conditions may struggle to lose weight despite following diet and exercise regimens, leading to frustration and health risks.

This chapter will explore how these conditions affect weight management, the importance of physician-supervised weight loss plans, and examples of effective treatments. We'll also include case studies to illustrate real-life scenarios where medical supervision was essential to safe and effective weight loss.

Hypothyroidism and Weight Gain

Hypothyroidism occurs when the thyroid gland does not produce enough thyroid hormones, which are critical for regulating metabolism. A sluggish metabolism often leads to weight gain and makes it difficult for individuals to lose weight, even with lifestyle changes. Other symptoms of hypothyroidism include fatigue, depression, and cold intolerance, which can further reduce a person's motivation to engage in physical activity or stick to a healthy eating plan.

Thyroid hormones—thyroxine (T4) and triiodothyronine (T3)—play a central role in metabolic processes, influencing how the body uses energy. When these hormones are deficient, energy expenditure decreases, and the body becomes more efficient at storing fat.

Case Study: The Impact of Hormone Therapy

A 35-year-old woman named Sarah struggled with weight gain despite maintaining a calorie-restricted diet and moderate exercise routine. She also experienced extreme fatigue and cold sensitivity. Blood tests revealed elevated thyroid-stimulating hormone (TSH) levels, indicating hypothyroidism. Her doctor prescribed levothyroxine, a synthetic version of T4, to bring her thyroid hormone levels back to normal.

After six months of consistent medication use and regular check-ups to adjust her dosage, Sarah's symptoms began to improve. Her energy levels increased, and she saw gradual weight loss as her metabolism stabilized. However, Sarah's physician emphasized the need for long-term medication use and regular monitoring, as improper dosing could hinder her progress.

Research supports that thyroid hormone replacement, when tailored to the individual, can help restore metabolic balance and facilitate weight loss in those with hypothyroidism . However, weight loss is often slower for individuals with this condition, and patience is key.

Polycystic Ovary Syndrome (PCOS) and Insulin Resistance

PCOS is a hormonal disorder that affects approximately 6-12% of women of reproductive age . It is characterized by elevated levels of androgens (male hormones), irregular menstrual cycles, and ovarian cysts. PCOS is commonly associated with insulin resistance, a condition in which the body's cells become less responsive to insulin, leading to elevated blood sugar levels and increased fat storage. As a result, women with PCOS often struggle with weight gain, especially around the abdomen.

Weight management is particularly difficult for individuals with PCOS because insulin resistance increases hunger, causes cravings for sugary foods, and promotes fat storage. Furthermore, elevated androgens can lead to muscle mass reduction, further complicating weight loss efforts.

Case Study: Addressing PCOS with a Physician-Supervised Plan

Megan, a 28-year-old woman with PCOS, had been trying to lose weight for several years without success. Despite following a low-calorie diet and exercising regularly, she continued to gain weight, especially around her midsection. Her doctor conducted tests that revealed insulin resistance associated with her PCOS.

Megan's physician created a comprehensive, physician-supervised weight loss plan that included:

- Metformin, a medication that improves insulin sensitivity, helping to lower blood sugar levels and reduce fat storage.
- A low glycemic index (GI) diet, emphasizing whole grains, lean proteins, and non-starchy vegetables to stabilize blood sugar.
- Strength training exercises to increase muscle mass, improve insulin sensitivity, and boost metabolism.

Within three months, Megan started seeing improvements in her blood sugar levels, reduced cravings, and gradual weight loss. Her doctor also recommended ongoing hormonal treatments and regular check-ups to monitor her condition and adjust her medication as needed.

Research supports the combination of Metformin and lifestyle changes as an effective way to manage both weight and insulin resistance in individuals with PCOS . Furthermore, a low-GI diet can help control blood sugar and reduce the risk of developing Type 2 diabetes, a common complication of PCOS.

Diabetes and Weight Management

Diabetes, particularly Type 2 diabetes, is closely linked to weight issues. Excess body fat, especially around the abdomen, contributes to insulin resistance, which impairs the body's ability to regulate blood sugar levels. As a result, individuals with Type 2 diabetes often find it difficult to lose weight, even though weight loss is crucial for managing the disease.

Weight loss can significantly improve insulin sensitivity, lower blood sugar levels, and reduce the need for diabetes medications. However, managing weight loss with diabetes can be tricky, as drastic dietary changes or increased physical activity can lead to hypoglycemia (dangerously low blood sugar levels) if not monitored carefully.

Case Study: Physician-Supervised Weight Loss for Diabetes

John, a 55-year-old man with Type 2 diabetes, had been struggling to lose weight for years. Despite his efforts to follow a diet and exercise plan, his weight remained stagnant, and his blood sugar levels were poorly controlled. After consulting with his endocrinologist, John was placed on a GLP-1 receptor agonist called semaglutide (brand name Ozempic), a medication that helps control blood sugar levels and promote weight loss by reducing appetite and slowing stomach emptying.

John's physician also created a personalized nutrition plan that focused on:

- Portion control and meal timing to prevent blood sugar spikes.
- Increasing protein and fiber intake to promote satiety and prevent overeating.
- A low-carb diet to stabilize blood sugar and encourage fat loss.

Over the course of a year, John lost 30 pounds, and his blood sugar levels were better controlled, reducing his need for additional diabetes medications. The weight loss also improved his energy levels and allowed him to engage in more physical activity, further improving his metabolic health.

Studies have shown that medications like GLP-1 receptor agonists not only help with blood sugar control but also aid in weight loss for individuals with diabetes . When combined with physician-supervised diet and exercise plans, these medications can be highly effective for weight management in diabetic patients.

The Importance of Physician-Supervised Weight Loss Plans

For individuals with medical conditions like hypothyroidism, PCOS, and diabetes, physician-supervised weight loss plans are essential. These conditions complicate weight loss efforts, requiring a more tailored approach that addresses the underlying medical issues while ensuring safety and effectiveness. Without medical supervision, individuals may attempt diets or exercise programs that exacerbate their condition, leading to health risks such as:

- Worsening hormonal imbalances.
- Severe hypoglycemia (for individuals with diabetes).
- Nutrient deficiencies that can worsen metabolic health.

Key Components of Physician-Supervised Weight Loss Plans

1. **Medical evaluation and diagnosis:** Proper diagnosis of underlying conditions like hypothyroidism, insulin resistance, or diabetes is crucial to creating an effective weight loss plan.
2. **Personalized medication regimens:** Medications like thyroid hormone replacements, Metformin, or GLP-1 receptor agonists should be tailored to the individual's needs and regularly adjusted.
3. **Dietary modifications:** Physicians may recommend specific diets, such as low-GI, low-carb, or high-protein diets, to stabilize blood sugar and support fat loss.
4. **Exercise guidance:** Supervised exercise plans that take into account the patient's medical condition are essential to ensure safe and effective physical activity.
5. **Ongoing monitoring:** Regular check-ups to monitor progress, adjust medications, and track weight loss are necessary to ensure long-term success.

Conclusion

Weight loss for individuals with medical conditions like hypothyroidism, PCOS, and diabetes is more complex than for those without these conditions. It requires specialized treatment, careful monitoring, and a tailored approach that addresses the underlying medical issues. Physician-supervised weight loss plans are essential for ensuring that patients lose weight safely and effectively while improving their overall health outcomes.

By combining medications, personalized diet plans, and regular exercise under the supervision of a healthcare provider, individuals with these medical conditions can achieve sustainable weight loss and better manage their health.

"The food you eat can either be the safest and most powerful form of medicine or the slowest form of poison."

– ANN WIGMORE

CHAPTER 9

Long-Term Weight Management
Sustaining Weight Loss and Promoting Longevity

Introduction

Achieving weight loss is only half the battle—long-term weight management is where the real challenge lies. Studies show that maintaining weight loss is often more difficult than the initial effort of losing weight. Without a structured plan and continuous lifestyle adjustments, many individuals regain the weight they worked so hard to lose, a phenomenon often referred to as weight cycling or yo-yo dieting. However, with the right strategies, long-term weight management is achievable and can lead to lasting improvements in overall health and longevity.

In this chapter, we will explore the most effective strategies for maintaining weight loss, including continuous monitoring, nutritional adjustments, and behavioral maintenance. We'll also discuss the role of Body Mass Index (BMI) as it relates to health and longevity, and the importance of maintaining a healthy weight over the lifespan.

Understanding Body Mass Index (BMI) and Health

Before diving into long-term weight management strategies, it's important to understand how Body Mass Index (BMI) relates to overall health. BMI is a simple formula used to estimate an individual's body fat based on their weight in relation to their height. The equation for BMI is:

According to the Centers for Disease Control and Prevention (CDC), BMI categories are as follows:

- Underweight: BMI below 18.5
- Normal weight: BMI 18.5 – 24.9
- Overweight: BMI 25 – 29.9
- Obese: BMI 30 or higher

While BMI is a useful screening tool, it doesn't directly measure body fat, and it can be influenced by factors like age, sex, and muscle mass. For example, older adults tend to lose muscle mass and may have a higher fat percentage even with a normal BMI, while athletes may have a higher BMI due to muscle rather than excess fat. Despite these limitations, BMI remains a valuable indicator for assessing health risks related to weight, such as heart disease, diabetes, and certain cancers.

Long-Term Weight Management: Why It Matters for Longevity

Maintaining a healthy weight is critical for longevity and quality of life. Research consistently shows that proper weight management can significantly reduce the risk of chronic diseases and extend life expectancy. A 2020 study published in the journal *The Lancet* found that individuals who maintained a healthy weight throughout adulthood were less likely to develop obesity-related illnesses, and they lived longer on average compared to those who experienced significant weight fluctuations.

Conversely, people who regain lost weight may be at a higher risk of developing conditions like metabolic syndrome, hypertension, and type 2 diabetes. This makes the practice of long-term weight management essential not only for maintaining a healthy appearance but also for promoting cardiovascular health, reducing inflammation, and improving metabolic function.

Strategies for Long-Term Weight Management

Achieving long-term weight management requires a combination of strategies that involve continuous monitoring, nutritional adjustments, and behavioral changes. These strategies are crucial to preventing weight regain and ensuring that individuals maintain their health gains over time.

1. Continuous Monitoring

Self-monitoring is one of the most effective tools for maintaining weight loss. Research published in *Obesity Reviews* highlights the importance of regular self-monitoring practices such as weighing yourself regularly, tracking your caloric intake, and monitoring physical activity. These strategies help individuals stay accountable and catch early signs of weight regain.

- **Regular weigh-ins:** Weighing yourself daily or weekly can help you track weight changes over time. Studies show that people who weigh themselves regularly are more likely to maintain their weight loss compared to those who do not. Regular weigh-ins also help individuals make quick adjustments to their diet and exercise routines if they notice weight creeping back up.

- **Food journals or apps:** Tracking your food intake through journals or mobile apps can help you maintain a calorie deficit or caloric balance after weight loss. Monitoring the types of foods you consume also ensures that you're sticking to a nutrient-dense diet rather than falling back into unhealthy eating patterns.

- **Activity tracking:** Monitoring physical activity with fitness trackers or apps allows you to ensure that you're meeting your exercise goals. Maintaining an active lifestyle is key to keeping the weight off, as regular physical activity boosts metabolism and burns calories.

65

2. Nutritional Adjustments

After reaching weight loss goals, many individuals mistakenly believe they can revert to old eating habits. However, nutritional adjustments are crucial for long-term weight management. Rather than viewing a diet as a temporary solution, it should be considered a lifestyle change that evolves over time to meet the body's needs.

> ▶ **Increase fiber intake:** High-fiber foods, such as fruits, vegetables, whole grains, and legumes, help keep you full longer and promote healthy digestion. Fiber also aids in blood sugar regulation, which can prevent weight regain.

> ▶ **Prioritize protein:** A high-protein diet is essential for maintaining muscle mass during weight maintenance. Protein helps preserve lean body mass, which is critical for keeping your metabolism high. Incorporating lean proteins such as chicken, turkey, fish, eggs, and plant-based options like tofu and lentils can help you maintain your weight over the long term.

> ▶ **Mindful eating:** Mindful eating practices, such as slowing down while eating and paying attention to hunger and fullness cues, can help prevent overeating and emotional eating. People who practice mindful eating are more likely to maintain their weight loss by avoiding impulsive food choices.

> ▶ **Portion control:** Even after reaching your target weight, it's important to practice portion control. Eating large portions, even of healthy foods, can lead to gradual weight gain. Monitoring portion sizes and avoiding calorie-dense foods like processed snacks, sugary beverages, and fried foods can prevent this.

3. Behavioral Maintenance

The psychological aspect of weight maintenance is just as important as the physical. Maintaining weight loss requires behavioral changes that help prevent old habits from resurfacing. Cognitive-behavioral techniques can be used to address the underlying causes of overeating and promote long-term behavioral change.

- ▶ **Goal setting:** Setting realistic, short-term goals helps to maintain motivation after weight loss. For example, setting goals for consistent exercise, healthy meal preparation, or hitting a daily step count can help keep weight management efforts on track.
- ▶ **Stress management:** Chronic stress can lead to overeating and weight regain through increased levels of cortisol, a hormone that promotes fat storage. Incorporating stress-reducing activities like yoga, meditation, or deep-breathing exercises can help prevent emotional eating and weight gain.
- ▶ **Social support:** Surrounding yourself with a supportive community—whether through weight loss groups, family, or friends—can improve adherence to weight management practices. Social support has been shown to increase motivation, provide accountability, and reduce feelings of isolation during weight maintenance efforts.

How BMI Changes with Age and Health Implications

As individuals age, BMI may change due to natural shifts in muscle mass and body composition. For example, older adults tend to lose muscle and gain fat, which can lead to an increase in BMI even if their overall body weight remains the same. It's important to note that sarcopenia, or the loss of muscle mass with age, can contribute to a higher body fat percentage, even in individuals with a normal BMI. This underscores the importance of maintaining muscle mass through strength training and a high-protein diet, especially as we age.

Maintaining a healthy BMI throughout life is crucial for reducing the risk of chronic diseases like heart disease, stroke, and diabetes. A higher BMI is associated with a greater risk of developing these conditions, while maintaining a BMI within the normal range can promote better metabolic health and extend lifespan. Research published in the *Journal of the American Medical Association (JAMA)* found that individuals with a BMI between 18.5 and 24.9 had the lowest risk of death from all causes, while those with a BMI over 30 had significantly higher mortality rates.

Weight Management and Longevity

Long-term weight management is not just about maintaining a specific number on the scale—it's about promoting overall health and longevity. Studies have consistently shown that individuals who maintain a healthy weight are more likely to live longer, healthier lives. For example, a large study published in *The New England Journal of Medicine* found that individuals who maintained a healthy weight had a lower risk of heart disease, diabetes, and cancer, leading to increased life expectancy.

Maintaining weight loss reduces inflammation, improves insulin sensitivity, and supports cardiovascular health, all of which contribute to a longer, healthier life. Additionally, individuals who maintain a healthy weight tend to experience improved quality of life, with more energy, better mobility, and a reduced risk of developing age-related diseases.

GLP-1 medications like semaglutide (Ozempic/Wegovy) have gained popularity for their effectiveness in weight loss, but they also play a critical role in long-term weight maintenance. After achieving significant weight loss, maintaining that new weight can be challenging due to metabolic adaptation, where the body naturally tries to regain the lost pounds. This is where GLP-1s shine.

GLP-1 medications work by regulating appetite and enhancing the feeling of fullness, making it easier to adhere to a healthy, reduced-calorie diet even after the initial weight loss. They also help manage insulin sensitivity and glucose levels, which is beneficial for preventing weight rebound, especially for those with insulin resistance or prediabetes.

For maintenance, it's important to pair GLP-1 use with continued lifestyle changes, such as regular physical activity and a balanced diet. These medications shouldn't be viewed as a standalone solution but rather as part of a holistic approach to long-term weight management. Physicians usually recommend a lower maintenance dose to reduce side effects while still supporting appetite control and metabolic health. Long-term adherence to GLP-1 therapy can help prevent weight regain and sustain the benefits of initial weight loss efforts.

Conclusion

Long-term weight management requires a multifaceted approach that includes continuous monitoring, nutritional adjustments, and behavioral changes. By focusing on these strategies, individuals can maintain their weight loss, improve overall health, and reduce the risk of chronic diseases that shorten lifespan. Maintaining a healthy BMI throughout life plays a critical role in promoting longevity, and the benefits of long-term weight management extend far beyond appearance—they impact the overall quality of life and life expectancy.

With the right tools, support, and mindset, sustainable weight management is not only possible but essential for a healthy, long life.

*"Movement is a medicine
for creating change in a
person's physical, emotional,
and mental states."*

– CAROL WELCH

CHAPTER 10

Insurance Coverage for Weight Loss Treatments

Navigating Health Insurance for Medications, Surgeries, and Counseling for Obesity

Introduction

Weight loss treatments, especially those aimed at addressing obesity and its related health conditions, can be life-changing. However, accessing these treatments often depends on insurance coverage. Whether it's prescription medications, bariatric surgeries, or nutritional counseling, navigating insurance policies and understanding what's covered can be a daunting process. In many cases, individuals may need to pay out of pocket for treatments, even when those treatments are essential for their health and well-being.

This chapter will explore how insurance plans address weight loss treatments, including the cost of medications like GLP-1 agonists (e.g., semaglutide, marketed as Ozempic and Wegovy), and bariatric surgery. We will also examine the financial implications for those who choose to self-pay for elective medical services, and why certain treatments, while not covered by insurance, are still critical for maintaining long-term health.

Insurance Coverage for Weight Loss Medications

Many individuals struggling with obesity turn to prescription medications to aid in weight loss. Among the most notable medications are GLP-1 receptor agonists, such as semaglutide, which have shown substantial efficacy in promoting weight loss. Originally developed for type 2 diabetes, GLP-1 medications like Ozempic, Wegovy, and tirzepatide (marketed as Mounjaro) have been approved for treating obesity due to their ability to regulate appetite and improve metabolic health.

Coverage of GLP-1 Medications

Insurance coverage for GLP-1 medications can be inconsistent. Some insurance providers view these drugs as medically necessary for individuals with diabetes but may not cover them for obesity treatment alone, even though the FDA has approved them for this purpose. For example, Ozempic is often covered by insurance for patients with diabetes, while Wegovy, which contains the same active ingredient, may not be covered unless a specific BMI threshold or comorbidity is met.

According to research from the Obesity Action Coalition, many health insurance plans categorize obesity medications as "lifestyle drugs," which means they may not be covered under standard policies unless the individual meets specific criteria, such as having a BMI over 30 or a BMI over 27 with at least one weight-related condition, like hypertension or heart disease.

Cost of GLP-1 Medications

For individuals without insurance coverage, the cost of GLP-1 medications can be prohibitively expensive. According to GoodRx, the average cash price for Ozempic is around $900-$1,000 per month in the United

States, while Wegovy costs approximately $1,300-$1,500 per month. Mounjaro, although still under evaluation for obesity treatment, is similarly priced. These high costs can make these medications inaccessible to many who need them.

Patients who do not qualify for insurance coverage or cannot afford the out-of-pocket costs may explore manufacturer savings programs or patient assistance programs, which can provide discounts or free medications based on income levels.

Insurance Coverage for Bariatric Surgery

Bariatric surgery, which includes procedures such as gastric bypass, sleeve gastrectomy, and lap band surgery, is often considered the most effective long-term treatment for severe obesity. Insurance coverage for these surgeries varies, but many plans will cover the cost if certain criteria are met.

Criteria for Coverage

Most insurance plans require patients to meet specific eligibility criteria to qualify for bariatric surgery coverage, such as:

- BMI of 40 or higher without comorbid conditions.
- BMI of 35 or higher with at least one obesity-related health condition, such as diabetes, sleep apnea, or heart disease.
- Documented failed attempts at losing weight through diet and exercise.
- Participation in a supervised weight loss program or nutritional counseling for a specified period (usually 3-6 months).

In addition to these requirements, insurance plans may require patients to undergo a psychological evaluation to ensure they are mentally prepared for the lifestyle changes that come with bariatric surgery.

Out-of-Pocket Costs for Bariatric Surgery

For those without insurance coverage or who are considering self-paying for bariatric surgery, the cost can be significant. According to the American Society for Metabolic and Bariatric Surgery (ASMBS), the average cost of gastric bypass surgery in the United States is between $20,000 and $25,000, while gastric sleeve surgery costs between $15,000 and $20,000. These figures vary based on the surgeon, facility, and geographic location.

Although self-paying for surgery is expensive, many patients choose this route due to the long-term health benefits. Bariatric surgery has been shown to significantly reduce the risk of chronic diseases like diabetes and heart disease, and in some cases, it can reverse type 2 diabetes entirely.

Insurance Coverage for Nutritional Counseling and Behavioral Therapy

Nutritional counseling and behavioral therapy are key components of a comprehensive weight loss plan, but they are often not fully covered by insurance. Many plans will cover a limited number of visits with a registered dietitian or behavioral therapist, particularly if these services are part of a weight loss surgery program.

However, for long-term weight management, patients may need ongoing counseling and support, which can result in additional out-of-pocket costs. Some insurance plans only cover nutritional counseling if the patient has a diagnosed medical condition, such as diabetes, rather than obesity alone. As a result, many individuals are forced to pay for these services themselves, even though they are critical for maintaining a healthy lifestyle.

Self-Paying for Elective Medical Services

For individuals who don't qualify for insurance coverage or whose plans don't cover specific treatments, self-paying for elective medical services is sometimes the only option. This can include paying out of pocket for weight loss medications, bariatric surgery, or non-covered therapies like counseling or alternative treatments.

Why Self-Pay Services Can Be Essential

While insurance companies often draw a strict line between what is medically necessary and what is elective, many self-pay services are still critical to overall health and quality of life. For example, weight loss medications like GLP-1 agonists may not be covered under standard insurance policies, but they can have profound health benefits, such as reducing the risk of cardiovascular disease, improving glycemic control, and boosting mental well-being.

Similarly, while bariatric surgery may seem like a drastic measure, it is medically necessary for many individuals who are at risk of life-threatening conditions due to severe obesity. Paying for these treatments out of pocket, while burdensome, is often the only way for individuals to regain control of their health and avoid complications associated with untreated obesity.

The Disconnect Between Insurance and Medical Necessity

One of the biggest challenges in accessing weight loss treatments is the disconnect between insurance policies and what medical professionals deem medically necessary. While insurance companies often view obesity treatments as cosmetic or elective, doctors understand that obesity is a chronic condition that requires medical intervention.

The American Medical Association (AMA) recognizes obesity as a disease, meaning that treatments aimed at weight loss are often not just about appearance—they are critical for preventing serious health conditions like heart disease, stroke, and diabetes. However, because obesity is still stigmatized, many insurance companies fail to provide adequate coverage for these treatments, leaving individuals to bear the financial burden.

Conclusion

Navigating the landscape of insurance coverage for weight loss treatments can be challenging, especially when policies vary so widely in terms of what they cover. Medications, surgery, and counseling for obesity are often treated as elective, even when they are necessary for long-term health. As a result, many patients must turn to self-paying for services that insurance won't cover, despite the fact that these treatments are essential to living a healthy life.

The financial strain of paying for GLP-1 medications, bariatric surgery, and ongoing counseling can be immense, but the health benefits—including reduced risk of chronic diseases and improved quality of life—make it a worthwhile investment for many. Until insurance policies evolve to recognize the full medical necessity of obesity treatments, individuals will need to weigh the costs and benefits of both covered and uncovered options as they pursue their weight loss journeys.

Here are 20 health tips for improving muscle mass, losing weight, and boosting energy levels:

▸ **Prioritize Protein Intake:** Protein helps build and repair muscles. Include lean sources like chicken, turkey, eggs, tofu, and beans in your diet.

▸ **Strength Train Regularly:** Engage in resistance training (weight lifting, bodyweight exercises) at least 3-4 times per week to build muscle and increase metabolism.

▸ **Stay Hydrated:** Dehydration can lead to fatigue. Drink plenty of water throughout the day to maintain energy and aid muscle recovery.

▸ **Eat Whole Foods:** Focus on whole, unprocessed foods like vegetables, fruits, whole grains, and lean proteins to fuel your body properly.

▸ **Consume Healthy Fats:** Fats from sources like avocado, nuts, and olive oil support hormone production and sustained energy.

▸ **Time Your Meals:** Eat small, balanced meals every 3-4 hours to keep your energy levels stable and metabolism active.

▸ **Include Complex Carbs:** Choose complex carbohydrates like brown rice, quinoa, and oats to fuel your workouts and support muscle growth.

▸ **Get Enough Sleep:** Aim for 7-9 hours of quality sleep per night to allow muscles to recover and keep energy levels high.

▸ **Supplement Wisely:** Consider supplements like creatine, whey protein, or BCAAs if you're struggling to meet protein goals or boost muscle recovery.

▸ **Incorporate HIIT:** High-intensity interval training (HIIT) burns fat efficiently while preserving muscle mass and increasing stamina.

▸ **Track Progress:** Keep a record of your workouts and nutrition to identify patterns and areas for improvement.

▸ **Don't Skip Breakfast:** Eating a nutrient-dense breakfast kickstarts your metabolism and energy levels for the day.

▸ **Focus on Fiber:** Fiber-rich foods like fruits, vegetables, and whole grains aid digestion and help control appetite.

▸ **Limit Sugary Foods:** Cut back on processed sugars and refined carbs, as they lead to energy crashes and weight gain.

▸ **Take Rest Days:** Give your muscles time to recover with rest days. Overtraining can lead to burnout and reduced progress.

▸ **Incorporate Compound Exercises:** Focus on exercises like squats, deadlifts, and bench presses that work multiple muscle groups at once.

▸ **Eat Post-Workout:** Consume a post-workout meal or snack with protein and carbs to promote muscle recovery and energy replenishment.

▸ **Stay Active Outside the Gym:** Increase daily activity through walking, cycling, or taking the stairs to burn extra calories.

▸ **Reduce Stress:** High cortisol levels from stress can hinder muscle growth and cause weight gain. Practice stress management techniques like meditation or yoga.

▸ **Set Realistic Goals:** Set achievable short- and long-term goals for muscle growth and weight loss to stay motivated and on track.

Made in the USA
Columbia, SC
08 November 2024

45811387R00057

DISCARD

Murder at Ford's Theatre